THE JOY OF VOLKSMARCHING
2ND EDITION

By

Mary Frances Going

Illustrated by

Mac Moody

To him who in the love of Nature holds Communion
with her visible forms, she speaks
A various language; for his gayer hours
She has a voice of gladness, and a smile,
And eloquence of beauty, and she glides
Into his darker musings, with a mild
And healing sympathy, that steals away
Their sharpness, ere he is aware.

from "Thanatopsis" by William Cullen Bryant

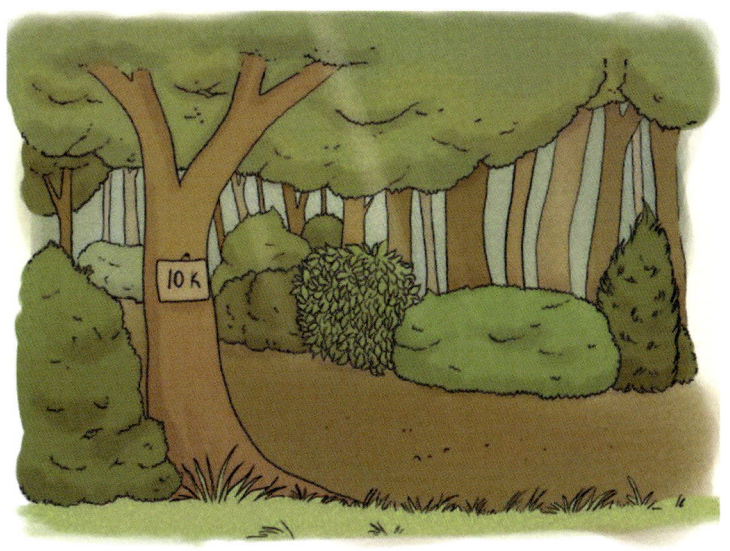

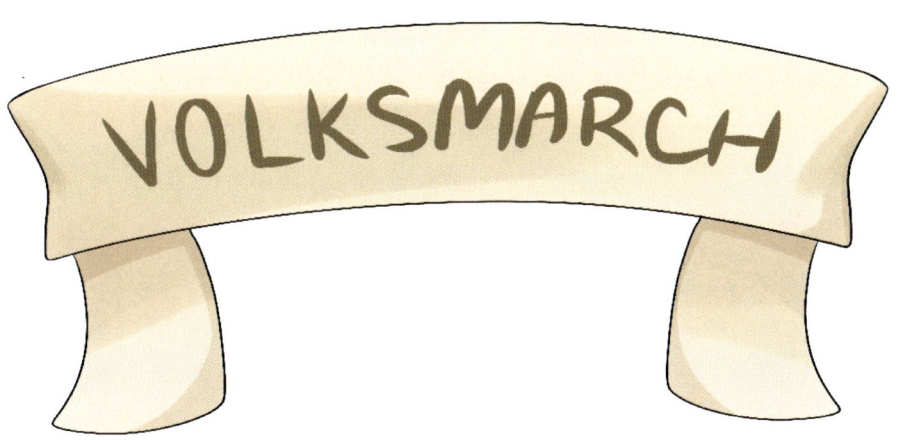

INTRODUCING – THE "VOLKSMARCH"

Out of bed at five in the morning, into old clothes (or new if you've decided to dress handsomely for the sport), socks and thick-soled walking shoes, a quick bite for breakfast, out of the house and into the car. Thus, a weekend morning often begins for thousands of volksmarchers all over Germany. You may have only a short distance to drive; or, if the volksmarch is farther away, an hour or two before you arrive at the starting point.

A "volksmarch," or "volkswanderung," to use the German expression, is simply a ten or twenty kilometer walk through the forests and fields and over the hills of the beautiful German countryside. These walks are planned either by German sports clubs or German communities and, more and more, by American military community volksmarching clubs. Some sponsor marathon marches of from thirty to forty-two kilometers. These are for the veteran marchers, but the great majority of walkers take the "ten." You may also graduate to a twenty kilometer when the 10K begins to seem too short. Ten kilometers is roughly six and one-fourth miles. The walks are registered with the IVV or DVV, Internationaler Volkssport Verband or the Deutschen Volkssportverbandes, and most of them are listed in a booklet published yearly. There are hundreds of them held throughout the year, primarily on weekends but occasionally on German holidays.

Brochures are published by the sponsoring club or community which list starting times, usually from 7:00 a.m. to 1:00 p.m., contain preregistration information and a description of the medals or other types of awards for which you pay a nominal fee and pick up when you've completed the walk. Sometimes the award is a plate, sometimes a desk or table ornament, sometimes a patch, but usually it is a medal. It may depict something seen on or near the walk – a castle, a bridge, a village. Sometimes a series of medals is offered over a period of three or four years with famous musicians, artists, political figures or other motifs depicted on them. Purchase of these awards is voluntary, and some veteran marchers have hundreds of them.

Cards also may be purchased for approximately $2.50. One may buy a card on which is stamped the number of walks he has taken; another card shows the number of kilometers walked. The beginner purchases a ten-volksmarch card and/or a one-hundred-kilometer card. When these are filled, a thirty march and a five-hundred-kilometer card are available, then a fifty march and a one thousand-kilometer card is offered, and so on.

Participants walk for various reasons. There are those who stroll, taking time to note the various beauties nature may have to offer—little clumps of mushrooms, wild flowers and berries, spider webs shining in the sun, small animals scurrying by, fruit laden trees, fern, and moss.

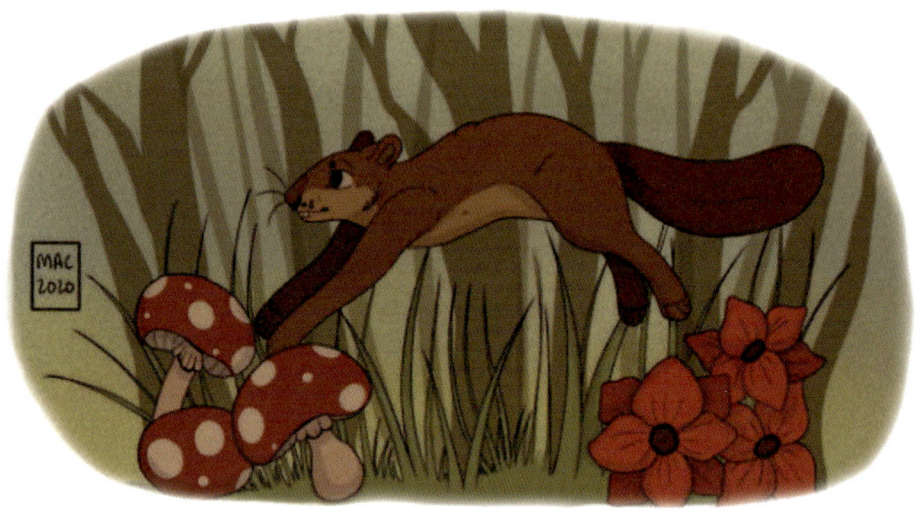

Others prefer a faster pace, timing themselves and taking pride in the shorter and shorter time it takes them to complete the walks. There are joggers on the trails, too; but for whatever reason they choose to walk, all the volksmarchers will tell you the benefits are worth the tired feet and sore muscles, for it is a relaxing and healthy sport.

In the following pages, the writer would like to take you along on a few delightful marches.

Thus, you may enjoy volksmarching vicariously, or perhaps you may wish to get out on the trails and learn for yourself the joys of walking, which thousands of Americans have discovered while on a tour of duty in the delightfully beautiful Deutschland.

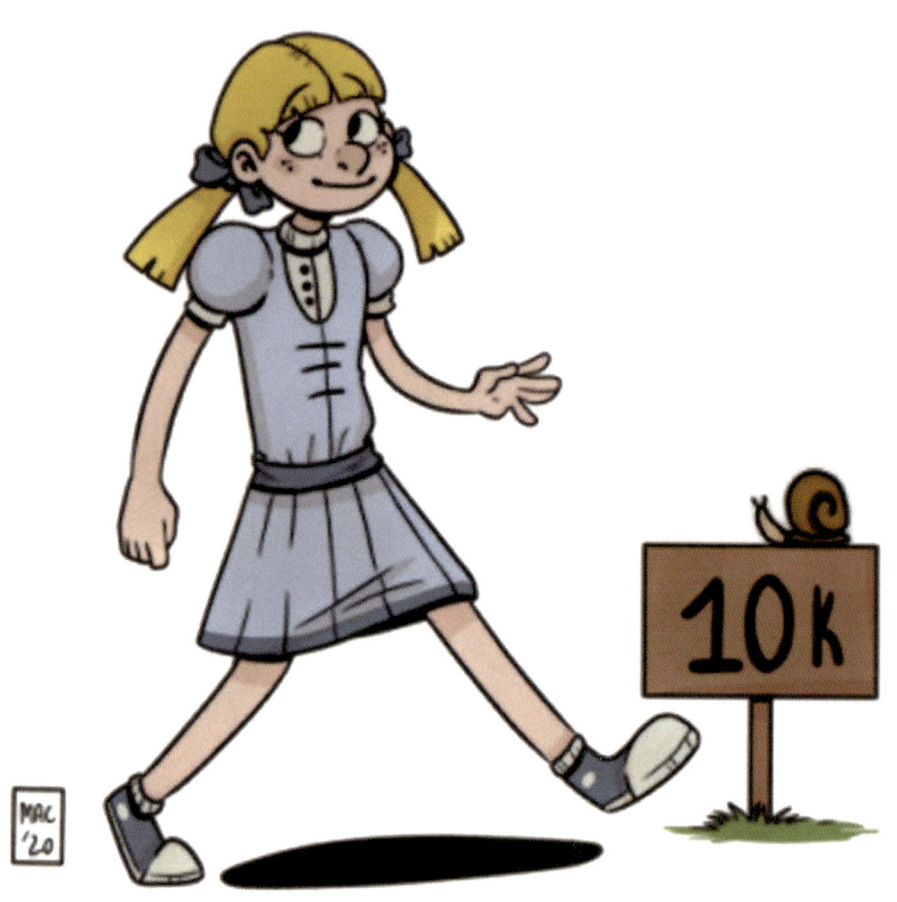

SCENTS, ODORS, SMELLS AND RHYTHM

Bruchsal, which is just down the road from Mannheim, was my destination one February morning. Off at 7:00 a.m., I was on the trail by 8:00. This was one of those days when the world was too much with me and I wanted solitude above all else.

Near the beginning of the walk, a German lady fell into step behind me. I tried speeding up, but she still managed somehow to remain only a short distance away. I finally sat down on a bench to let her get far ahead of me. As I sat there, it occurred to me that this was a ridiculous territorial body language on my part – the lady had been alone and making only the small sound of footsteps on the forest path. (My, Mary Frances, you are uptight today!) Still I continued to sit until I was sure she was enough ahead that I would not overtake her.

A beautiful volksmarch this was not. I remember it chiefly for smells. It led at its inception down by the railroad tracks and past warehouses. The odor of pine emanated from a lumber yard – a pleasing smell, reminiscent of East

Texas forests and Christmas trees.

Although it was not raining when we entered the forest, it had been earlier, and the sky was still overcast. The odor of wet leaves greeted me, and I liked that wet forest scent. Three young men in blue sweatsuits went jogging by. Listening and watching the fascinating rhythmical sounds of their feet and motions of their bodies until they were out of sight, a brief and foolish notion passed through my mind – "That had some of the elements of the dance. I would call it the 'jog trot.'"

It had begun to rain once more, and I put up my umbrella. From a distance and behind me, I heard singing and soon a group of French soldiers went by. Now and then they would break into song. As they passed, one of them tapped the top of my umbrella with a brochure as he sang and smiled. I was charmed and returned his greeting with a smile of my own.

We finished the march in a high-rise area where people watched us from their windows. One little girl – five-ish – smiled and waved vigorously. I smiled, too, as gas odors came up from a sewer, and I reflected on the incongruity of it all – the pleasant scents of pine and wet forest when I began and was uptight and irritable; the sewer smell at the end when I had relaxed and the events of the march had mellowed my mood.

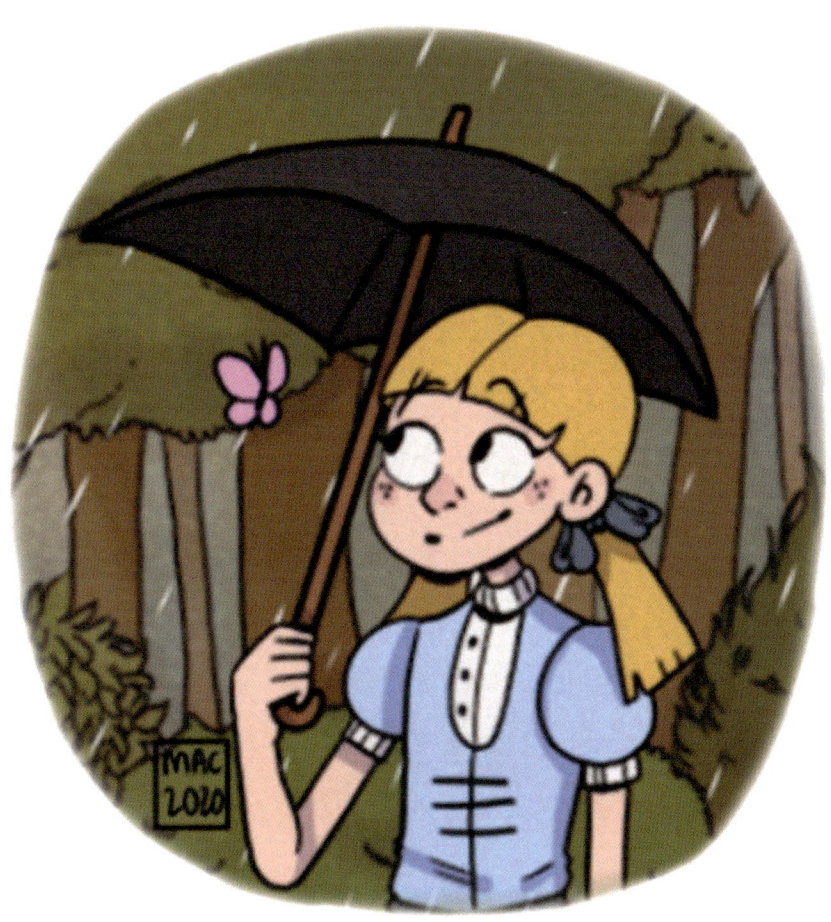

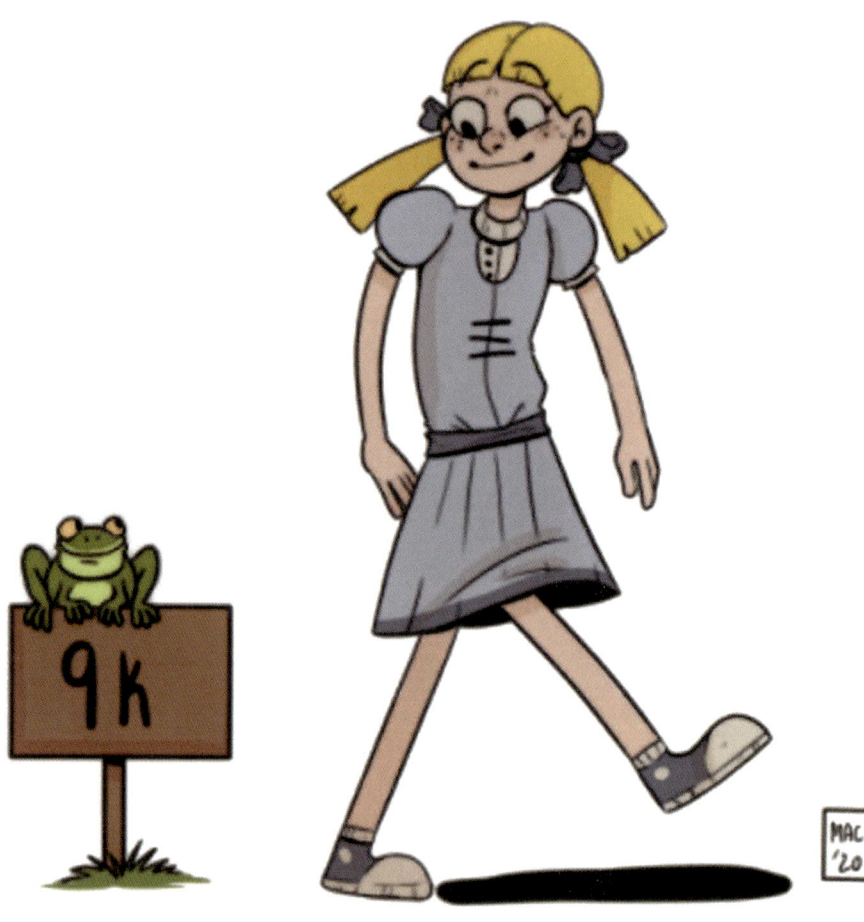

OUCH!   GROAN!   OOOOOOOOO!

Today in Eichelberg, not far from Bruchsal, I walked a "twenty," and my overtaxed muscles are complaining even after a hot bath for relief. I left home early; and, having arrived before the crowd, was on the trail by 8 a.m. It led first through a new residential area, and I stopped a time or two to admire the architecture of several houses. At one of them I was amused at the antics of a tiny little girl who peered at the marchers, then quickly ran to hide. Venturing out to peek once more, she remained poised for flight, and when her courage failed, off she went again. A young boy – eightish – passed me and smiled with "Guten Morgen." (Good morning.)

Shortly I came upon an artificial lake and sat upon one of the benches beside it, taking time to jot down a few observations in my notebook. The place was full of early morning quiet, and I listened to soft bird sounds, the rushing of water through a pump, the town clock as it chimed the quarter hour. I didn't feel too well physically and emotionally was a macramé of knots from the week's minor upsetting events. Gradually, the peacefulness of the place and the moment stole into my spirits, and I felt better by the time I arose from the bench and resumed the march.

Having encircled the lake, I entered the woods. Here already was a control point with a fire glowing under crossed sticks, laughter and loud talk, and marchers' dogs barking at one another. One little dog kept whining and pulling on the leash. Perhaps, like me, he wanted to get away from human noises and into the peace of the woods. I had a bouillon which was being offered in place of the usual tea, then marched on.

After several kilometers through the woods, the path came out upon a river. Here, an elegant white swan floated around an island, in the middle of which was built a small animal shelter where another swan and a few ducks were reposing. Before crossing a rustic bridge, which led to a walk down the other side of the river, I noticed a playground built for children out of logs and other natural forest materials. "The Germans really are a 'master race' in some respects," I thought, "in cleanliness for one and in preservation of forest beauty for another."

Church bells from the nearby village to which we had walked heralded my decision to take the twenty-kilometer trail, for it was just beyond the river that the paths divided. I wasn't tired, and the day was a bit gray, but not bad, so I decided on the longer walk.

The "ten" had been flat, but now the trail rose upward toward vineyards and arbors above the village. Here were villagers doing March things – trimming and attaching grape vines to wires. One worker had affixed a transistor radio to a pole and was listening as he clipped. Some were trimming fruit trees, while others gathered the trimmings and burned them in bonfires. A man with a tub in his arms went along splashing water onto the ground, immediately followed by another who tossed to the ground on either side of him what appeared to be seeds.

All of this was interesting but soon gave way to rolling hills, which while lovely to look at, meant straining tired muscles up one hill and down another. After about six hours of walking, I arrived at the "ziel," purchased a "wein schorle" (wine and mineral water), and a steak sandwich, collapsed on a bench and munched away while watching other tired marchers come dragging in.

When the man stamped my book, he wrote in "21 K's" instead of "20." That one was the "K" that broke the marcher's back.

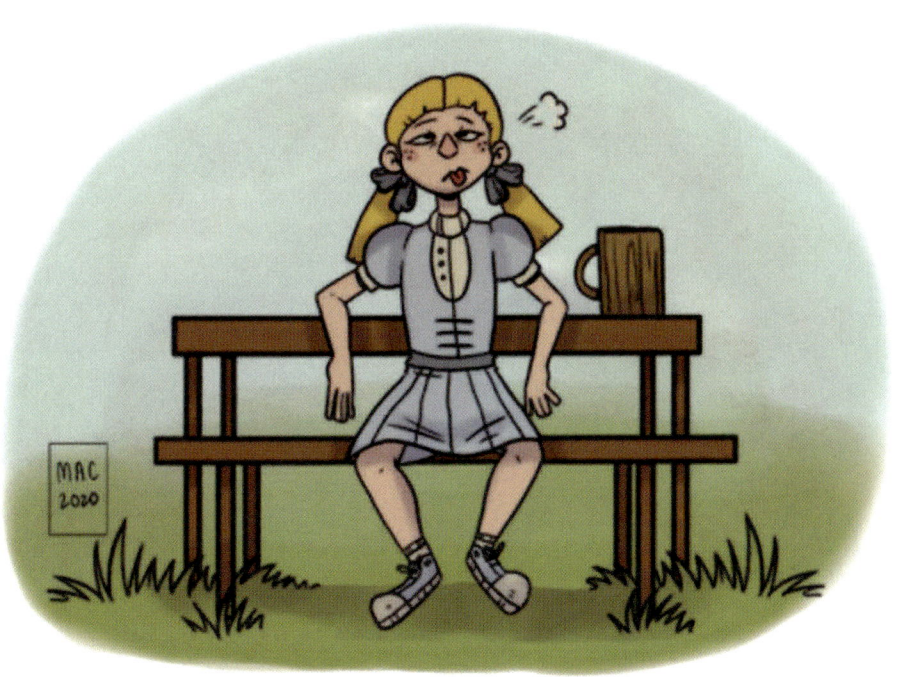

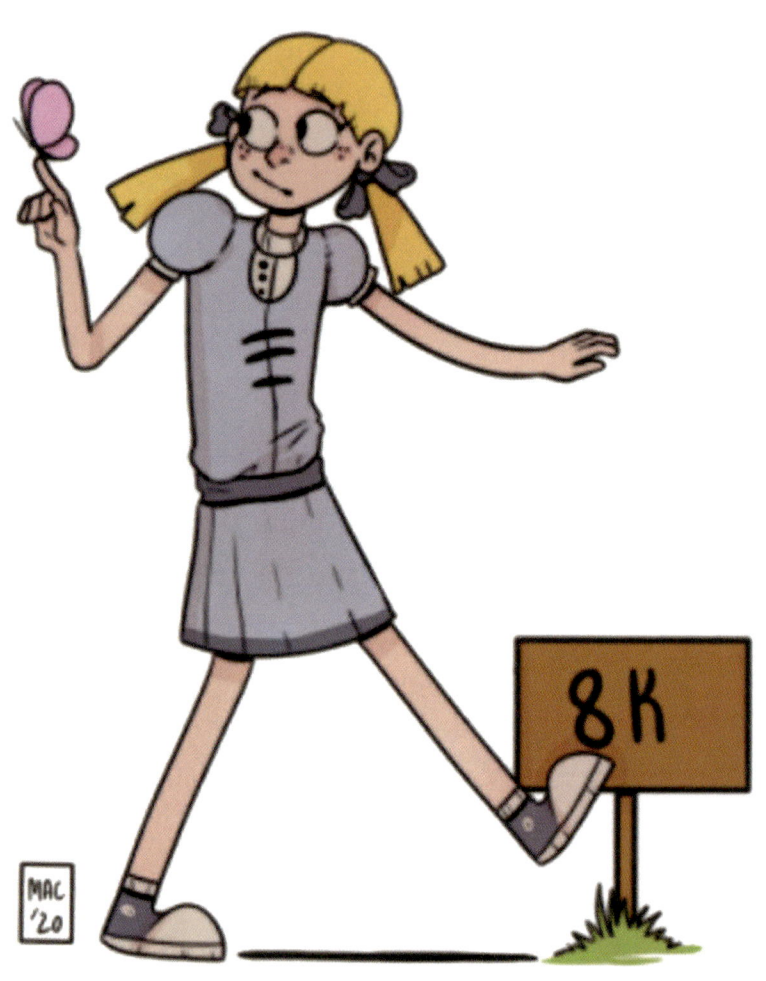

MISTY, MOISTY, MUDDY MARCHES

A dedicated volksmarcher must be prepared to endure all sorts and conditions of weather.

One particular Saturday, I toyed with the idea of doing two ten-kilometer marches. With this in mind, I started from home around 6 a.m., hoping to reach Langenlonsheim, near Bad Kreuznach, not later than 7:30 a.m. Surrounded by a pea-soup fog, I made a wrong turn and found myself in the town of Frankenthal. I lost about one-half hour there trying to wend an uncertain way back to the autobahn. Once more on the chartered course, I drove to Bad Kreuznach, where, invariably, I get lost, and today was no exception. Bad "K" is a small town, and a nice one, but for a stranger, poorly marked; and I lost another half-hour searching for signs to Langenlonsheim. After stopping several times for directions, suffering a number of well-deserved oaths and gestures from other drivers, I found the way and arrived at Langenlonsheim within ten minutes.

Quickly completing the volksmarching preliminaries, I struck out on the trail. It was still early morning, and the muddy path led through vineyards and into the forest. The rain-like precipitation from the trees was so heavy that I raised my umbrella. Everything was outlined in fog, and those who passed took on a strange, other-worldly appearance as they moved into the distance. The mud on the path became softer, my feet began sinking deeper and deeper, and my dark blue pants were soon spattered with mud. The fog cleared before the march was finished, but the day was still wet and dreary. At the "ziel," I met Darla Graczyk, who invited me to join her in another volksmarch near Kaiserslautern. I thanked her but declined as I had already decided to drive on to Obernhof near Koblenz.

Having lost that hour earlier in the day, I rushed down the highway, seeking Obernhof, which was also difficult to find, and I simply guessed my way to it, arriving just before the registration closed.

This walk began, continued and ended in mud. It led through beautiful countryside, by waterfalls and icefalls, over rustic bridges crossing brooklets and running beside a rushing stream; but I was so busy pulling one foot out of the mud and watching it sink again while teetering from side to side in a desperate effort to balance that I could not appreciate the beauty and charm of the place. More than once I slipped and almost landed sitting up in mud. Thank heavens I had my cane!

At the control point – another muddy pig bath – a man said to me in German, "It will take a long time to clean the shoes, no?"

"Yes!"

The following week, Dottie Van Norman reported a telephone conversation she had with Darla who said, "It's a good thing Mary Frances didn't go with me because the second volksmarch I took was very muddy!"

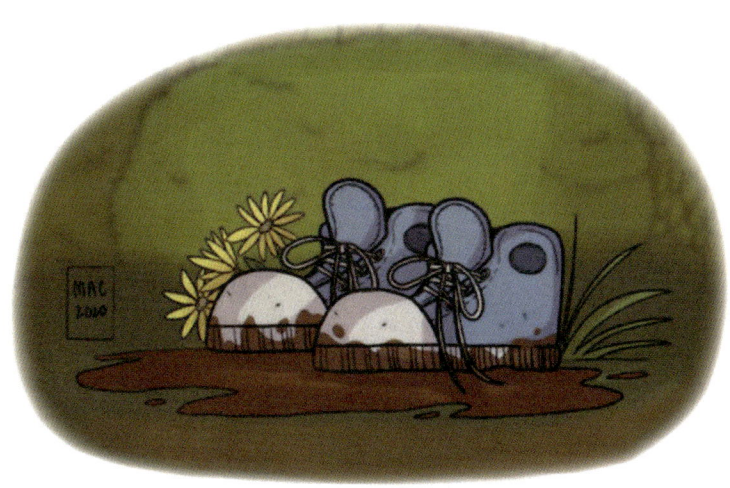

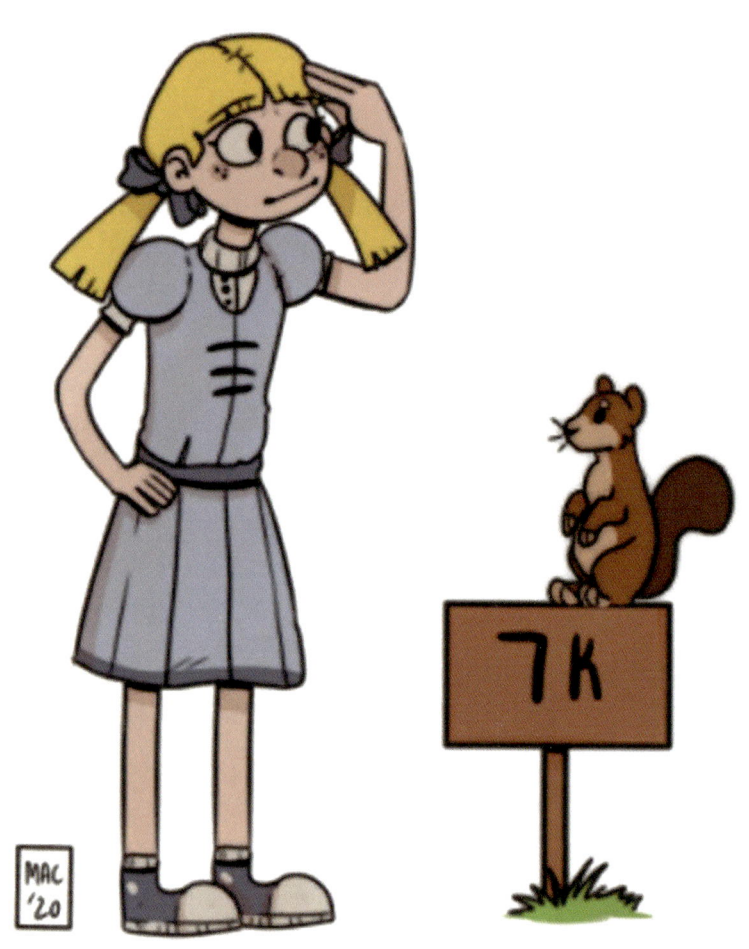

COW CHIPS AND SPIDER WEBS

Plankenstadt, September 17, 1978

One September Sunday I took a stroll among fruit-bearing orchards and through thickets of young birch where sunlight through the leaves dappled the toadstools and feathery ferns covering the shaded ground. My companion was Linda Montgomery, a charming young teacher from North Carolina and new to our school.

Although it was a beautiful day, it became a bit warm, and my feet were swelling. I complained to Linda; and overhearing me, a Canadian marcher just ahead turned around and advised me that soaking swollen feet in cow chips was an old Canadian remedy. I replied that I would rush right home and try it – though finding the necessary chips in my little metropolitan suburb was going to present something of a problem.

While resting at a control point, I described to Linda a beautiful dew-dusted spider web, sparkling and shining in the early sunlight that Chris Lins and I had found on a march. Chris wanted a picture, so we stepped off the path to get a bit closer. It was a perfect web, and we stood for

21

a moment just admiring its beauty. The light rays, bending as they touched the dew, added a suggestion of color to this little gem of nature. As Chris tried to get the web into focus, she moved the limb upon which it was hanging, and it fell and disintegrated. We both had a dismayed feeling that something beautiful had been destroyed.

Leaving the control, Linda and I continued on our way toward the end of the march. When for some reason I was bemoaning the fact of my growing old, Linda said in her fresh, sweet, young way, "Oh, Mary Frances, you aren't growing old if you can still get excited over a spider web!"

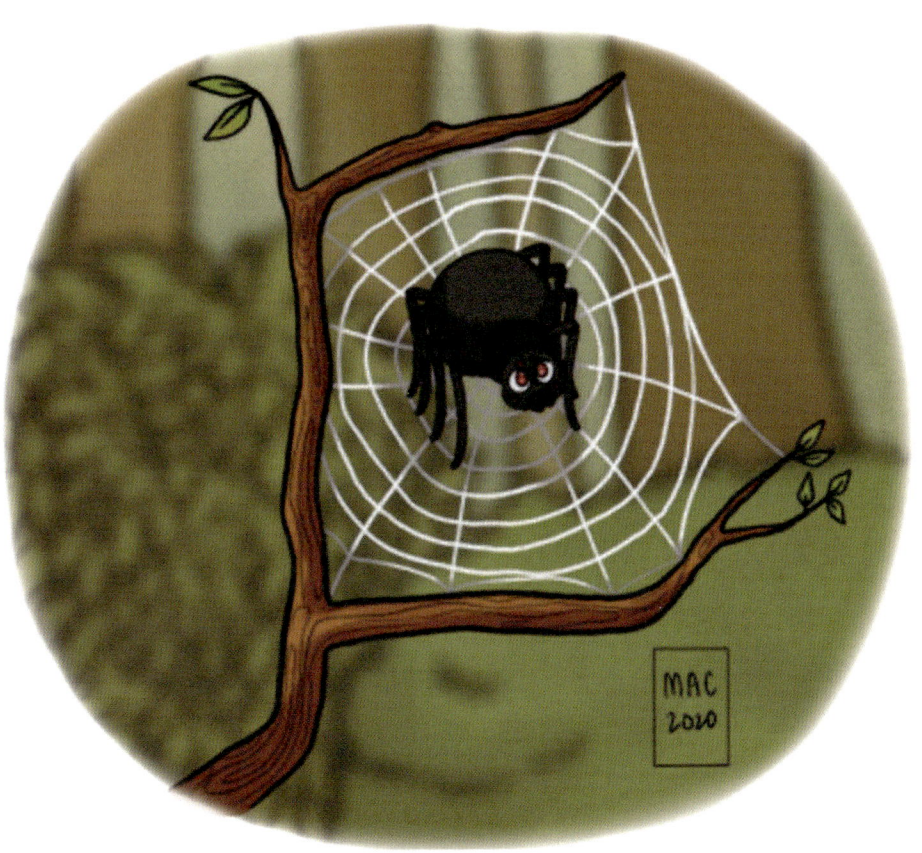

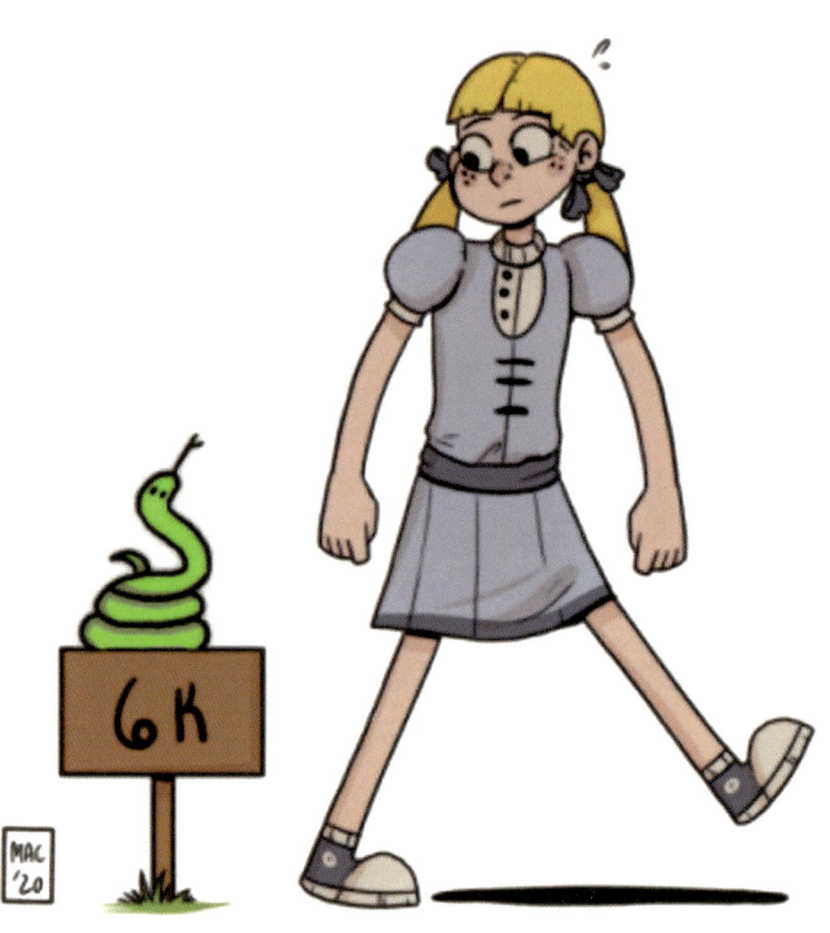

NOT A DAY – AN EXPERIENCE

Kaiserslautern, March 24, 1979

The title of this vignette must be credited to a friend, Mary Erickson, who, once on a lovely sunny drive through Alsatian France, uttered a beautiful thought – "This wasn't a day, it was an experience!" How perfectly that describes this day's volksmarch in Kaiserslautern.

Arising about five a.m., I looked out the bay window of my apartment to check the weather and saw a beautiful and perfect crescent moon. Although it was not yet light enough to know what the day would be, the streets were dry and all looked clear.

After I had eaten a light breakfast, my friends, Dottie and Brenda, arrived, and we set off for Kaiserslautern. It was chilly, with frost on the cars and breaths visible on the air. We bought our cards, made our routine trip to the "Damen" and set out. Although cold, we had such an exhilarated feeling of well-being – the French call it, "bien etre," – we were glad to be alive.

I explained to my friends that through volksmarching I was growing interested in learning about plants and flowers and even thought bird-watching could be fascinating – all those things that I looked on as a little crazy when I was much younger. Dottie suggested that perhaps I was just growing a little crazy. I admitted, though reluctantly, that that was a distinct possibility.

Dottie, the real volksmarcher among us, was a bit incapacitated with a strained ligament in her foot, so she was hobbling along with a cane. Brenda wasn't an experienced volksmarcher, so she wasn't taking the trail at too fast a pace. I took off from my friends for a while, therefore, and made my way through the woods and up and down hills at a fairly rapid clip. Eventually, I heard a woodpecker – a new sound for me as I had never heard one before. I sat down on a log at the side of the trail and just listened to his intermittent knocking. I decided I might write an ode, "On Hearing the First Woodpecker in Spring."

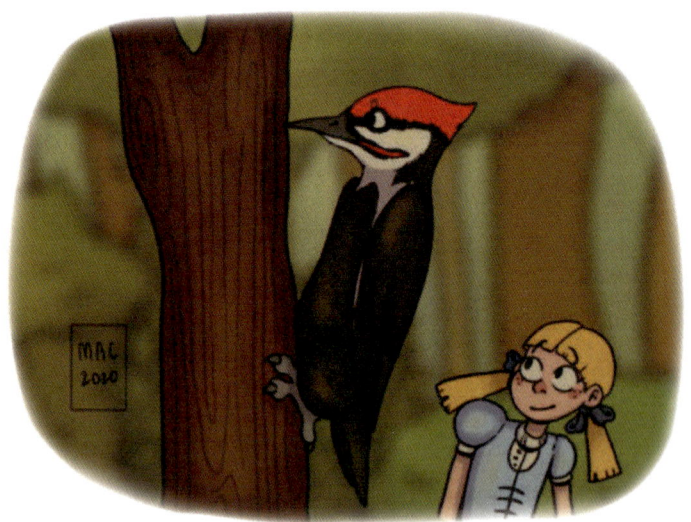

Darla Graczyk met us at the control. She was finishing the thirty-kilometer walk. While she and I walked back to the ziel together, she related the story of a friend who just the week before had died on the trail while they were volksmarching together. Our conversation reminded me of a march the week before where I heard a bird twittering incessantly and very, very loudly so that it attracted my attention as it flew high over the trail. "He's as joyful over spring and nice weather as I am," I thought. But then suddenly, he dropped straight to the ground. Whether his twittering indicated pain, or whether he was, as Brenda suggested later, like the thorn bird who experiences a moment of great ecstasy just before dying, I'll never know, but I hope that he was like the thorn bird for I think it is a lovely way to die.

Blessed all along the march with a beautiful sun, a cloudless sky, a greening forest and the company of good friends – we had, not a day, but an experience!

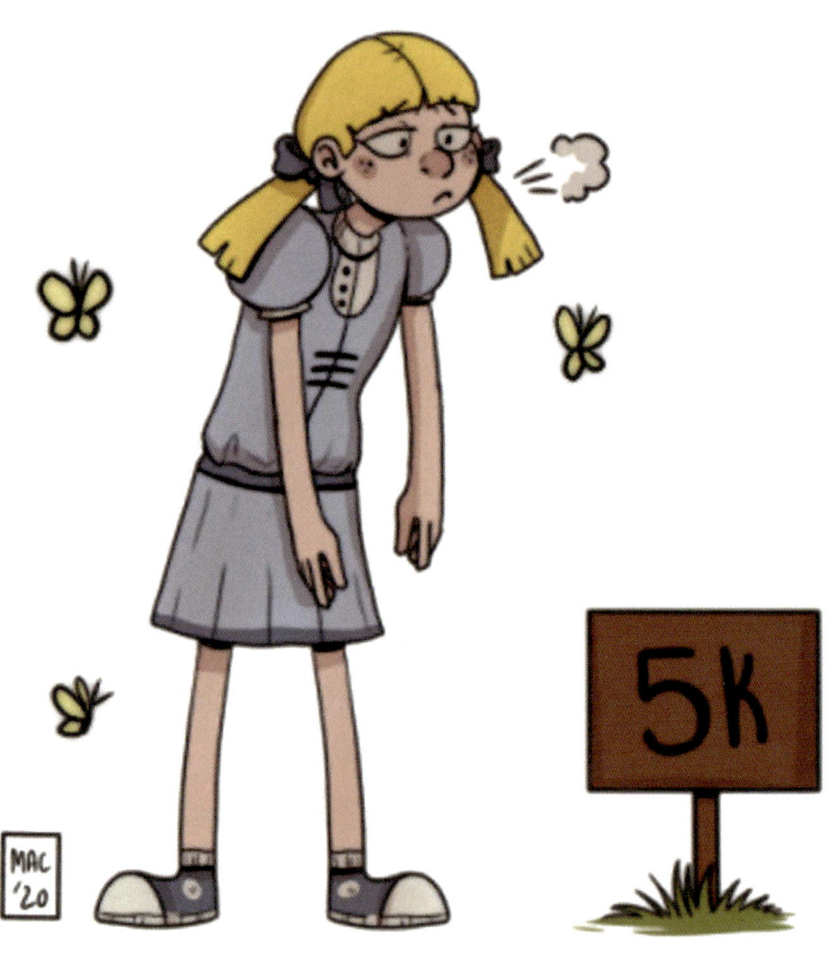

S-E-P-T-E-M-B-E-R

Weissach, September 16, 1978

Some volksmarches will be remembered
simply for their beauty. This was one. The sun
was shining; the air was cool; the fields and forests
still summer green. There were few marchers,
perhaps because it was Saturday and many
Germans were at work, but that was an added
bonus for I find luxury in the absence of crowds.
Not long after starting, I came upon a plum tree by
the side of the road bending low under its burden
of ripe plums.

Not having eaten breakfast, and feeling like
a guilty youngster, I picked about ten and
proceeded to eat them all. They were juicy and
sweet, and I relished each bite.

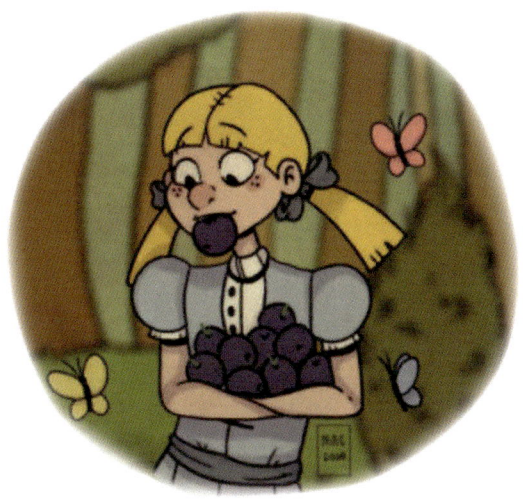

I ate as I walked, and the path soon led past a tree laden with ripe pears which I couldn't reach or might have had one of those, too. Nearby one fellow had stepped off the path and was picking and eating wild blackberries. If I hadn't been so "plum-full," I would have joined him.

Farther along, having passed an apple orchard with fruit-ladened trees, the path meandered into open fields where tractors were pulling various farm implements for harvesting the crops. Nothing outstanding here, but it all spelled "September."

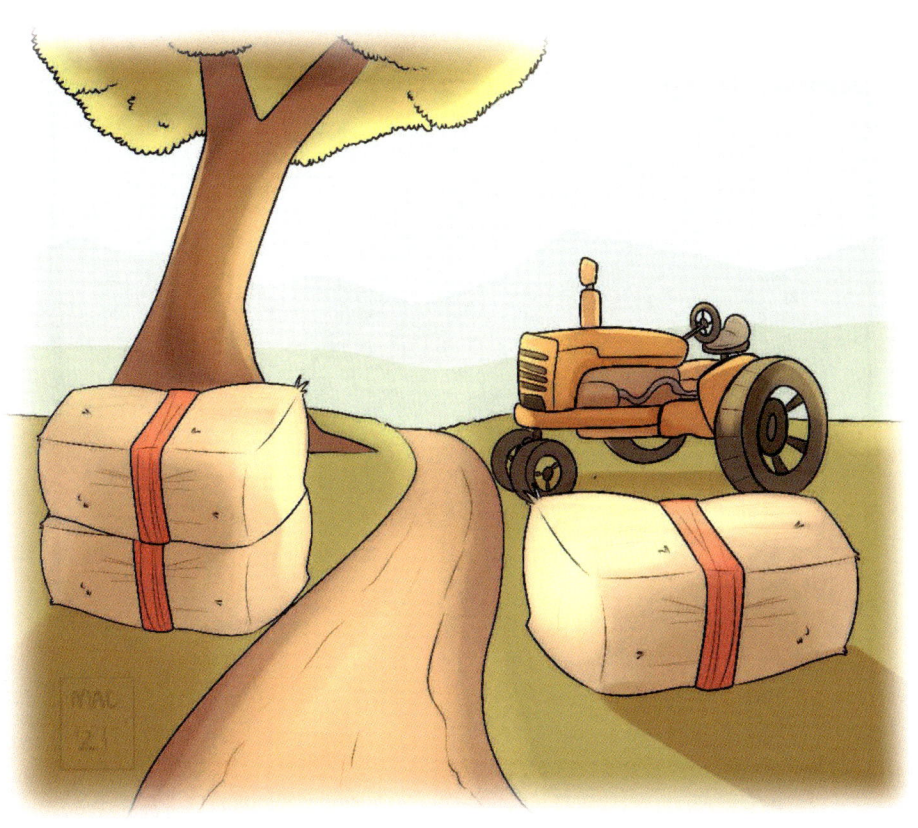

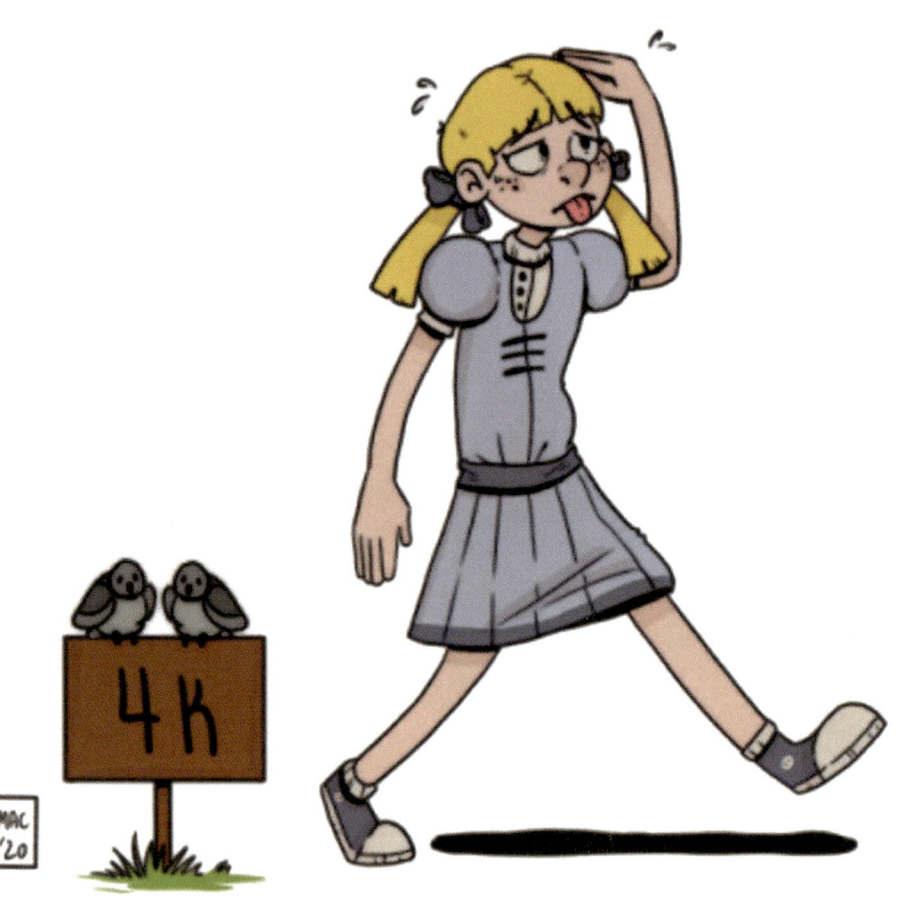

A WALK IN THE ODENWALD FOREST

This walk began in mist, but as the day and the march grew older, the mist lifted little by little and nature gradually removed her veil to show us what beauty she had prepared.

The very tall trees of the forest guided my eyes upward where they feasted upon a cathedral of autumn color. Now and then a leaf would drop and float down toward me, and I could imagine a voice whispering gaily, "Here you are, dearie, a lovely one just for you."

The path ran far from the ruins of Burg Rodenstein – year 1634, and I stepped off the path to get a better view. Situated in the midst of fog, the old castle had an other-worldly appearance; and, in my imagination, I could envision lords and ladies of a bygone era wandering around the grounds. I looked at my feet and wondered if one of that grand nobility had stood in this very spot and viewed the castle then as I was doing now.

Farther along, I stopped once again to watch and listen to a brooklet making its way down the hillside. The loud and incessant conversation of two ladies invaded my "sound territory," and for a few minutes, I could hear nothing else. They passed quickly, however, and once again, I enjoyed the brooklet's gurgled song.

After a rather long and steep climb, I sat on the end of a log to rest and to enjoy the parade of marchers going by. Some walked very deliberately, never looking to left or right; some were so engrossed in conversation that they were oblivious to everything around them; still others jogged by, sweating from every pore – their facial expressions akin to pain. The poet in me was offended, and I resisted the impulse to stand upon my log and declaim, "Oh, stop and be still for a moment or two! You are walking in such beauty and completely unaware!"

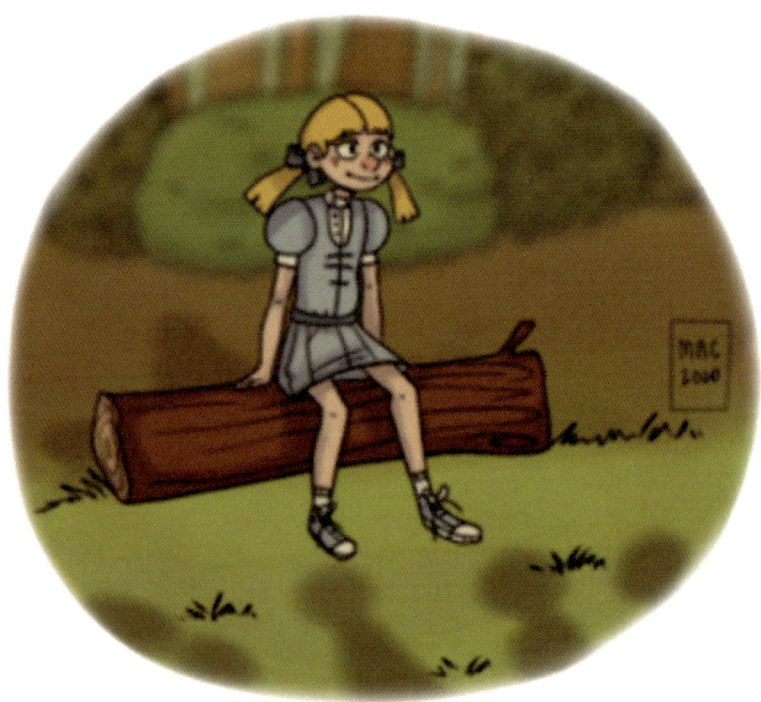

I trudged on, loving the soft, foot-soothing feeling of a pine needle path and the dew diamonds adorning the trees. Later, back at the clubhouse, sipping a wine schorle (wine mixed with mineral water), eating a sandwich and recording a few observations in my notebook, I thought again of the runners and the joggers and all the other marchers rushing along the paths, and I was reminded of a quip I heard once concerning the Louvre: "Pausing one minute in front of each item, it would take you thirty-nine years to go through the museum – but you could do it in fifteen minutes on roller skates."

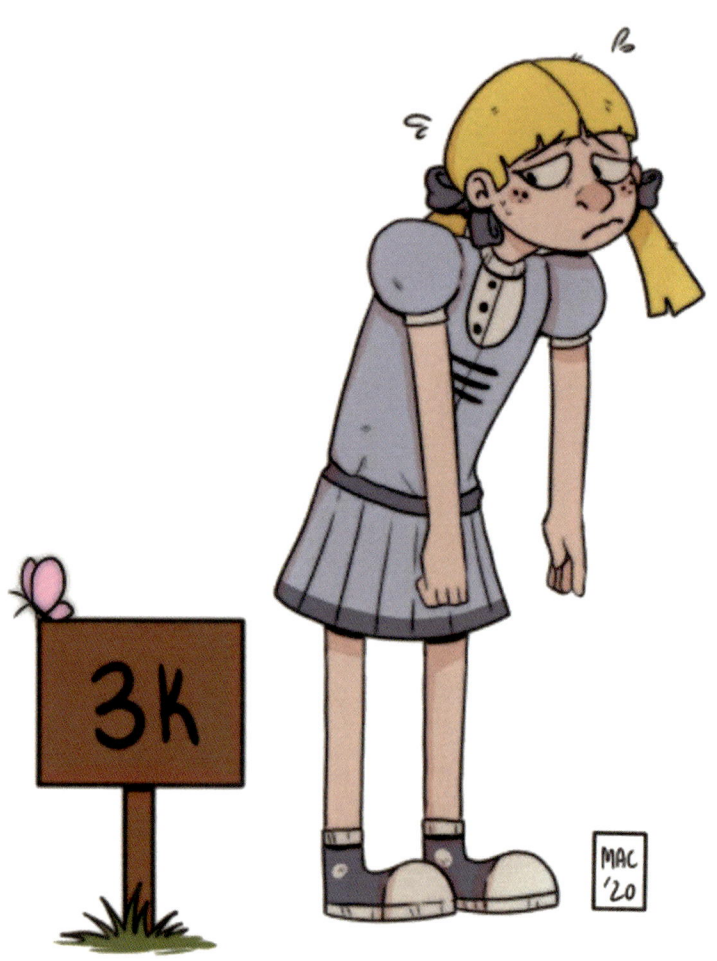

LEAVES DROPPING AND EAVESDROPPING

Ittlingen, October 21, 1978

At the beginning of this march, I passed a farm with a gaggle of very large geese. I saw one pinching another with his beak while his victim thrashed about uttering screams and cries and trying to escape. Being a city gal and ignorant in the ways of geese, I wondered if this were merely goose-play and not serious or whether the one was fed up with the other's infidelity or annoying, irritating ways. Was the victim really in pain, or just playing along in the age-old mating game? Perhaps even a country gal wouldn't know.

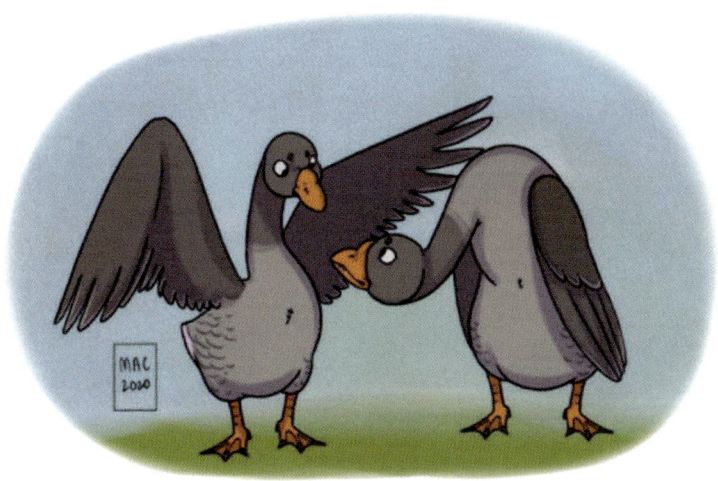

I overheard an interesting discussion of volksmarching by some Americans just ahead of me on the trail; and since by now I was definitely gathering materials for these vignettes, I cocked my ears and eavesdropped shamelessly. A GI was describing a four-day march of forty kilometers per day. He said, "If you do it in formation, you get to wear a patch on your fatigues." That's ninety-six miles! It occurred to me that they'd have to stretch the "patched fatigues" over my coffin if I took that march – in or out of formation.

There were two controls on the "ten." I had tea at the first, and at the second, a delicious steak sandwich and a "wein schorle" (a refreshing mixture of wine and mineral water). I kept quite a rapid pace until the second control, having done a bit of running, then took the last few kilometers leisurely.

Although it had been a month since I had walked, I wasn't terribly tired, but took no chances on sore muscles and went to Miramar (an indoor spa) and the sauna soon after arriving home. That completed some badly needed rejuvenation, and I felt great afterward!

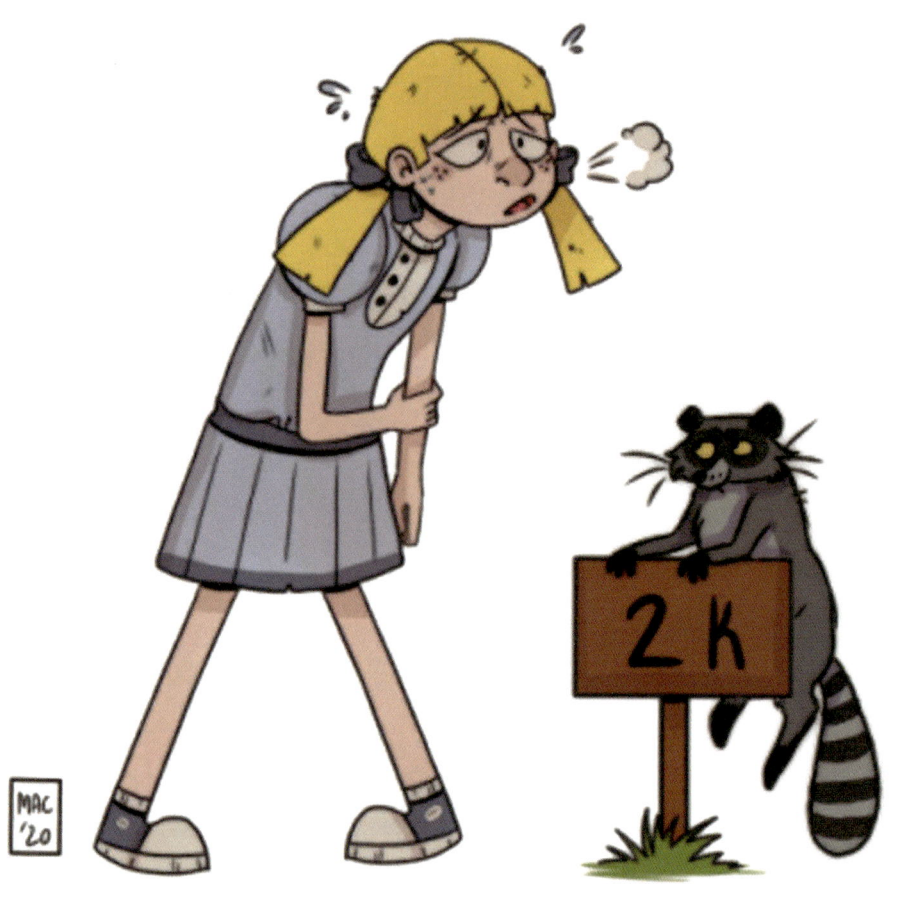

40

A VOLKSWALLOW IN MUDDY CLAY

Mud is muddy and messy enough, but when it is mixed with clay, it is impossible! An hour-long drive to Wiesbaden-Erbenheim in pouring rain should have forewarned me. The American woman's "bad" in answer to my queries concerning the condition of the trail should have deterred me, but I am a "cockeyed optimist" and so moved bravely out and on.

Three kilometers later I reached a control point, convinced that my American advisor must have been new to the sport if she found this trail "bad." I sipped my gluhwein and rested, smiling smugly as I prided myself on being an experienced marcher who had made conquest of many less-desirable trails. After a ten-minute respite, I continued with confidence.

Five minutes away, the path led across a field, and it was then that my folly became apparent, for the trail became a sty of slippery, muddy clay. Once in the mess, there was no escaping. Sometimes in a forest, one can leave a muddy path and walk through the woods on the side. No such easy solution was available here, for on each side of this path there was simply more of the same.

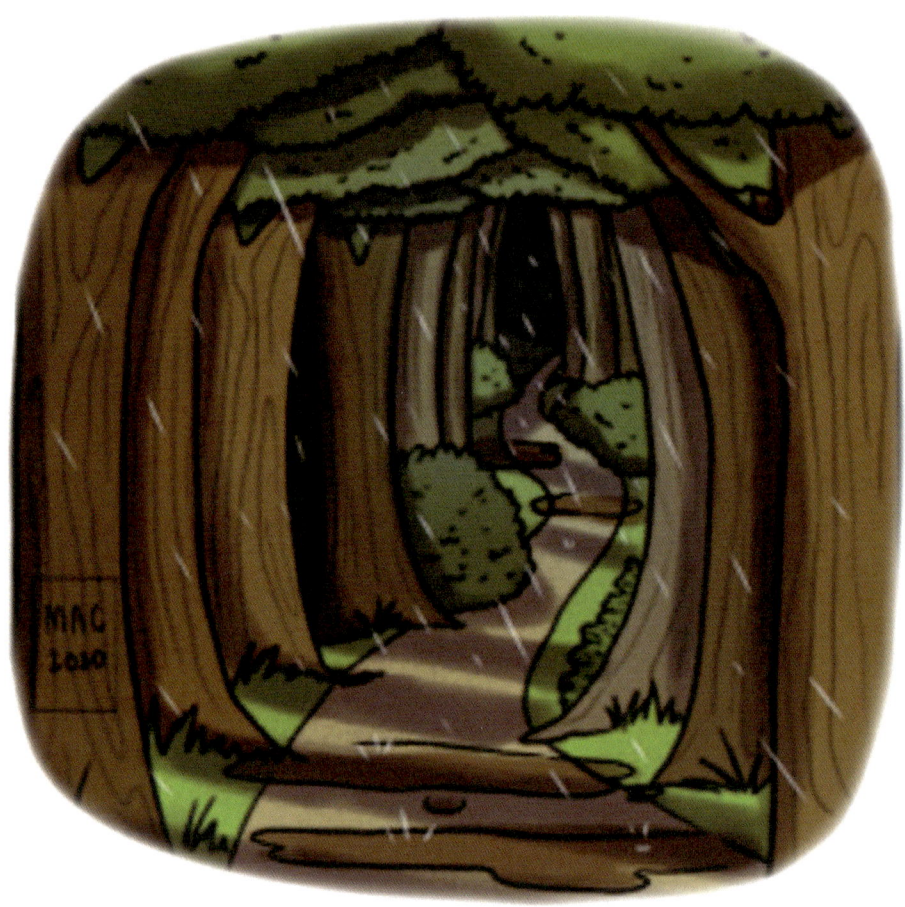

The wind was blowing a gale, making balancing difficult, and my feet were coming out of my shoes which were sticking in the clay. What I finally dreaded and feared most happened. I slipped and fell. My pants, cape, walking stick, umbrella and gloves were all a soggy, muddy mess. Some gracious people helped me up, although they were having as much difficulty as I. On we went struggling and fighting to be free of the mire. Eventually we were, and I trudged on, muddy and miserable. I had planned to take the fifteen-kilometer walk, and when the paths divided and I could see in the distance marchers on the "ten" going through a field of mud similar to the one we had just departed, I decided to take a chance on the "fifteen" being better. It went through several more muddy places but none as bad as the first. When I finally reached the "ziel," the end of the march, a man looked at me sympathetically and said, "I can see you've been on it." I smiled ruefully and countered, "In it!"

I drove home in a blizzard, fortunately without a mishap. Later, sitting in the cleanliness and warmth of my apartment, I could laugh at the comment of a German man on the trail who, observing my condition, asked, "Do you know the difference between a muddy volksmarch and this one?" I grimaced and said, "No." His reply, "There isn't any!"

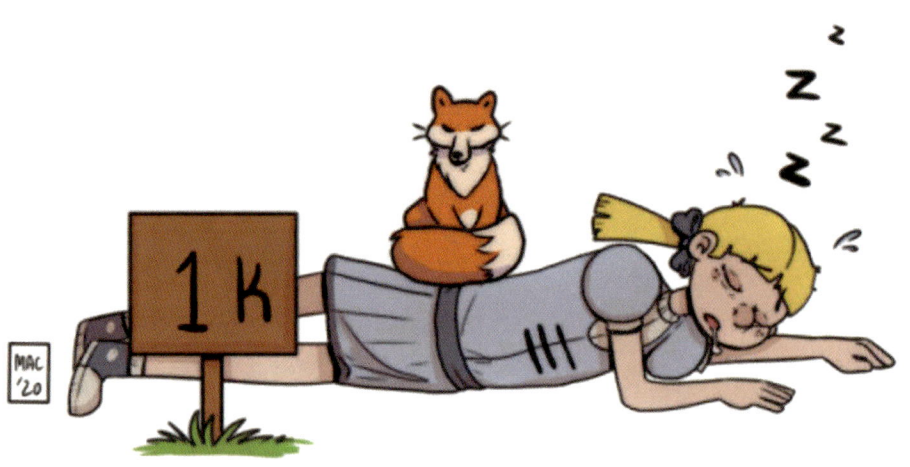

A MOO MOO HERE AND A MOO MOO THERE

Spring, 1978

I have recorded neither the exact date nor place of this volksmarch, but one word stands out as identification – "cows."

Dottie Van Norman and I did two "tens" that day, and I have no notes on the first. Sometimes a brochure advertises a "night" walk. Actually, it is an early evening march starting about 4 o'clock. Because the days in later Spring and Summer remain light until 9:30 or 10:00, one can easily do one of these marches before dark. There are, on rare occasions, "torchlight marches" which extend after dark and on which one carries a flashlight.

But back to the cow pastures. Our evening walk was indeed beside many groups of grazing bovines. What was remarkable was all the "mooing" going on. It sounded like "cow talk" as one seemed to answer another, and I asked my farm friend, Dottie, if they could be "be-mooing" the fact that their keepers had not come to milk and bed them so they could get on with a pleasant evening in the barn. She had no answer.

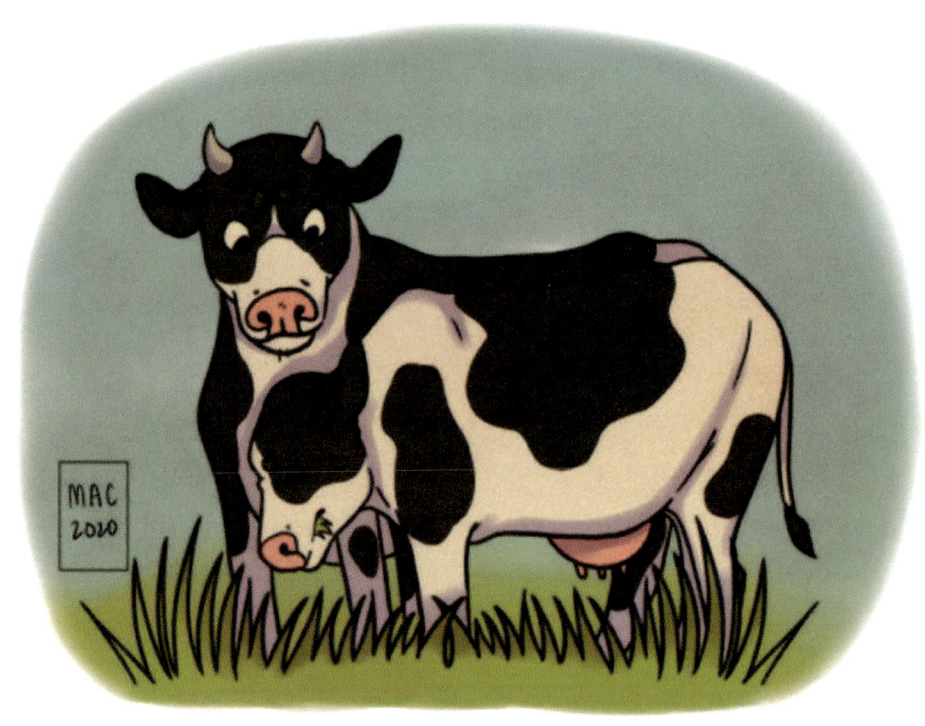

As we walked in silence listening to this cow concerto, my thoughts began to resemble a conversation which went something like this: "How now, Brown Cow?" "Well, you know, I have an easy life. I don't have to work, and I just stand around all day grazing with the other cows while nature manufactures the milk within me." "Ah, yes, Brown Cow, would that we all had it so easy!" "But, consider this, Human Being, I am not free. I must depend on someone to take me to and from the pasture. I must wait for someone to milk me, to feed me, to bring the vet when I'm ailing." "You are right, Brown Cow, freedom may make life harder, but freedom is better."

If cows could really talk, it might make for some very good listening.

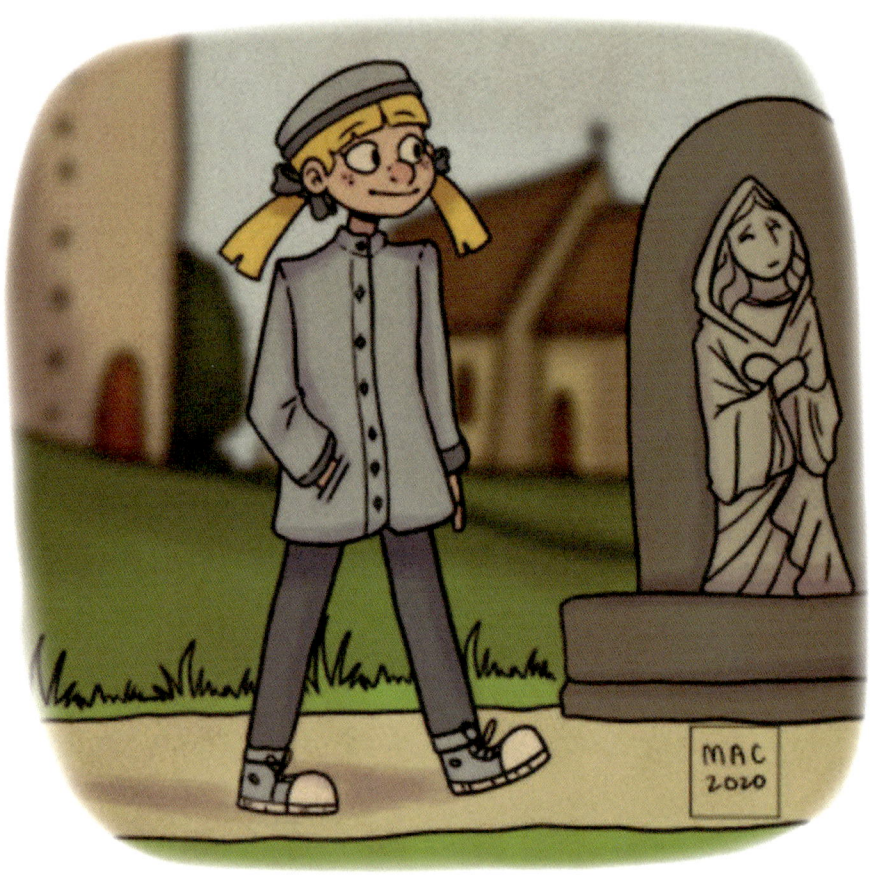

SUNDAY, SUNDAY!

Butenbach – near Waldmohr, October 22, 1978

An old church square, a small white statue of the Virgin and a stone lamp resting beneath an encased wooden crucifix – all seemed very apropos for the beginning of a Sunday morning pilgrimage through the woods.

Attaining the path by climbing a set of stone steps, I was busy praying that I wouldn't freeze to death as it was sprinkling slightly and I hadn't dressed for a cold communion with nature. My prayer was soon answered as the path began a long, steep ascent. Beginning to feel warm, I right away shed my rain cap and gloves and put them inside my zippered jacket which made a very convenient carry-all in spite of the fact that I must have looked stuffed – which indeed I was.

Somewhere along the way I was amused to see two beautiful palomino ponies and three black cows, who, instead of frolicking and munching in the meadow, stood side by side behind a fence, facing the path. The city girl couldn't say, but the would-be philosopher-poet wondered if they, like humans, wanted a bit of companionship – or perhaps were just watching the zoo go by.

Although the forests were beautiful, the leaves were dropping with every gentle breath of the breeze. At one point a brisk wind swept through the trees and showered the path and me with red and gold. Feeling blessed by nature, I thanked her silently, and she acknowledged my gratitude with another colorful blessing. This is the most beautiful time of year in the forests, but one feels a poignant sadness knowing that all of this beauty is short-lived and but a glorious goodbye to summer. Soon the trees will be bare; and unless whitened by a coverlet of snow, in a few short weeks the forest will present a bleak and colorless setting for those who seek its solitude.

The end of the walk led into a deep ravine spanned by three wooden bridges which the path traversed. At the side of the last stood a wrought-iron cross – a fitting end, I thought, for a Sunday walk in the woods.

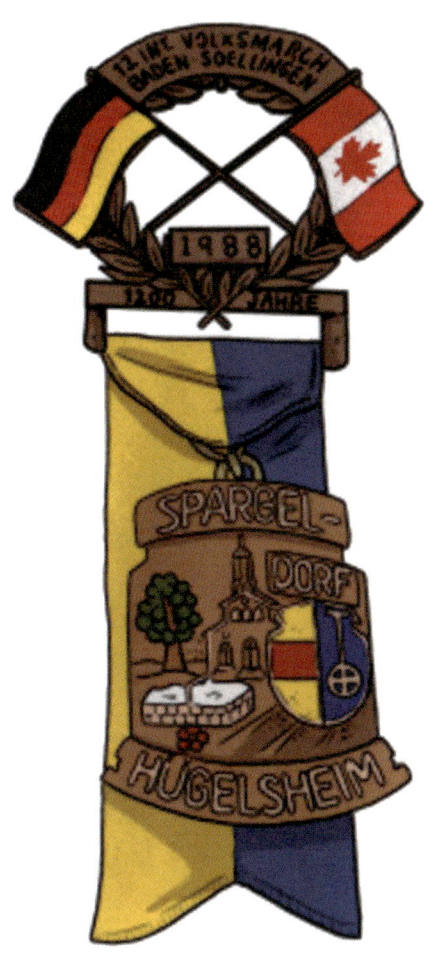

MARY FRANCES GOING

Born in Port Arthur, Texas, Mary Frances Going graduated with two degrees in music from the University of Texas at Austin. Following graduation, Mary Frances spent many years teaching music to the children of American servicemen and servicewomen in France and Germany. It was while she was in Germany that Mary Frances discovered the joy of volksmarching. A non-competitive form of fitness walking, volksmarching first rose in popularity in Europe in the late 1960s. Mary Frances joined other devotees of the sport, walking five, ten and sometimes twenty kilometers each weekend through the scenic pastoral areas outside Manheim, Germany. When she returned from Europe and moved to Colorado Springs, Mary Frances found that many communities had local volksmarching groups founded by military families who had brought the love of the sport back home with them. At age 96 and now living in the Texas Hill Country, Mary Frances credits the years of weekend volksmarching with her long life and good health. For more information or to find a local club near you, see the American Volkssport Association (aka "America's Walking Club") website at AVA.org.

Illustrator Mac Moody is an aspiring young artist from Kerrville, Texas. Currently a sophomore at Angelo State University in San Angelo, Texas, Mac notes that art has always been incredibly important in her life from her earliest years. After earning her Bachelor of Arts degree, she plans to combine teaching art with doing freelance art on commission.